# ACUPUNCTURE POINTS

# QUICK GUIDE

**Also by Deborah Bleecker**

*Insomnia Relief*
*Natural Back Pain Solutions*
*Acupuncture Points Handbook*

This book is an excerpt of *Acupuncture Points Handbook*. It is a practical reference for the points that are most commonly used in the clinic.

# ACUPUNCTURE POINTS

# QUICK GUIDE

Deborah Bleecker, LAc, MSOM

# Disclaimer

This book contains the opinions and ideas of the author. It is intended to provide helpful and informative material on the subjects addressed. It is sold with the understanding that the author and publisher are not engaged in rendering medical, health, psychological or any other type of advice or services in the book. If the reader needs personal, medical, health, or other assistance or advice, a competent professional should be consulted.

The author and publisher disclaim any responsibility for any liability, loss or risk, either personal or otherwise that occurs as a consequence, directly or indirectly, of the use and application of the contents of this book.

# Contents

## Acupuncture Meridians and Points

## Extra Points

Ba Feng – Eight Winds
Ba Xie – Eight Pathogens
Hua Tuo Jia Ji – Paravertebral points
Xi Yan – Eyes of the knee
Yao Tong Xue – Lumbar pain points
Zi Gong – Uterus point

# Introduction

How does acupuncture work?

If you want to understand acupuncture, you need to know how each point works. Once you determine which organ is not functioning well, you treat that organ via the points that affect it.

For stomach issues, you can use Stomach 36 to regulate the stomach. For emotional issues, such as anxiety, and insomnia, you can treat the Heart via Heart 7. Kidney problems can be treated by stimulating the points on the Kidney meridian, such as Kidney 3, 6, or 7. By regulating the organs and restoring normal function, the root cause is treated, and the health issue can be resolved.

Although there are over 400 acupuncture points commonly listed in textbooks, the truth is that there are points that are used most frequently. Points like Stomach 36, which improves digestion, boosts energy levels, and regulates the immune system.

If you would like a book that includes over 400 acupuncture points, *Acupuncture Points Handbook*, is the best option. If you would like to know which points are the most commonly used, this book is it. The points in this book are the ones that most acupuncture patients will experience.

Although I have included information on Chinese medicine theory, it is not necessary that you understand Chinese medicine to benefit from this book. Each point is fully explained in both Chinese medicine theory, and Western medicine theory.

**Meridian Images**

The meridian images that are at the beginning of each meridian section include the point numbers. Due to the number of points in some areas, it is not always possible to number all the points on those meridian images. For more precise locations, see the individual points. I have also included images showing how to locate some of the more commonly used points.

**Acupressure**

If you would like to treat yourself with acupressure, I have included an explanation of how to treat yourself effectively. Please be aware that there is misinformation online. Always ask for the credentials of the person who is giving you advice. The problem is not that you would be harmed by advice that is not correct, but that you would conclude that acupressure does not work.

**See a Licensed Acupuncturist, an LAc**

If you would like to get acupuncture, it is best to find a Licensed Acupuncturist. In order to be licensed by the state, an acupuncturist must have graduated from an acupuncture school, which is a graduate level program. A Licensed Acupuncturist has a degree in Oriental Medicine.

My degree is a Master of Science in Oriental Medicine, or MSOM. Other acupuncturists might have different types of degrees, but the goal is to find someone who studied Chinese medicine for three or four years in school. This will ensure you get the best care possible. Oriental medicine includes all aspects of Chinese medicine, such as Chinese herbal medicine, acupuncture, Gua Sha, cupping, moxibustion, and Tui Na, which is Chinese therapeutic massage.

## Point Functions

I have chosen the most commonly used point functions and symptoms associated with each point. I compiled information from multiple sources. I have included how the points function in Chinese medicine terms if it is important to know. In most cases the functions are explained using modern medicine terminology.

## Bulleted Lists for Major Acupuncture Points

The most commonly used acupuncture points are usually the points that have the most indications, or functions. I have indicated which points are commonly used by making the indication list a bulleted list.

The major points often have many functions and are much stronger than other points on the meridian. There are some points that are rarely used. They might be used to treat pain, by combining them with other points on the meridian, but they are less likely to be used to treat internal ailments.

## Unbelievable Acupuncture

You might find it hard to believe that the points do what they are listed as doing. You are not alone. It is always surprising and even after 20 years of studying acupuncture, I continue to learn new points, and new ways to use the points I have known about for 20 years.

Chinese medicine is a very rich medicine. After over 2,000 years of use, it continues to grow. Although modern research has yet to be able to explain how acupuncture works, it has been shown to work as the primary form of medicine in China for thousands of years. It is able to heal things that modern medicine cannot, because it helps the body to heal itself. Acupuncture restores healthy function to the body. It helps your body to heal itself. If you have ever been healthy, your body knows how to heal itself. It just needs a stimulus to encourage it to heal.

## Point Location

Most acupuncture points are located on both sides of the body. You can treat either side. Some points are located in the middle of the body, such as the Ren meridian, or the Du meridian, and there are special points that are treated on one side only.

## Acupuncture during Pregnancy

There are points that are not to be used during pregnancy. You will find that different sources cite different points. The most commonly listed points to avoid during pregnancy are Spleen 6, Large Intestine 4, Ren 4, Bladder 31, 32, 33, 34, Gallbladder 21, and Bladder 60. These points are contraindicated during pregnancy, which means they should be avoided during pregnancy.

Although getting acupuncture during pregnancy will help the mother have a very calm baby, these points are typically avoided unless the mother is ready to give birth. In addition to using acupressure on Pericardium 6 to treat nausea during pregnancy, the point Bladder 67 is used to turn the baby when it is in a breech position.

Although some points should not be used during pregnancy, it is highly unlikely there would be a problem. In fact, some acupuncturists specialize in treating women during pregnancy, to relieve problems associated with pregnancy, or to relieve stress and improve energy levels. I do not recommend acupressure for pregnant women, without professional advice from an acupuncturist. Please see a Licensed Acupuncturist for help.

**Naming of Meridians**
Each meridian has a name. Some of the meridians are commonly referred to by their English names, and others by their Chinese names, such as the Ren meridian. The Ren meridian is also called the Conception Vessel. The Du meridian is also called the Governing Vessel. The meridian names tell you what organs they connect to, but that does not mean that is all they do. Each meridian is interconnected to other meridians. It is virtually impossible to treat one isolated ailment. Each point has so many functions, and the meridians are interconnected.

You will see several different names for a meridian. Other names include channel, and vessel. A meridian is a pathway in the body. When you stimulate an acupuncture point, it stimulates better circulation in the treated meridian, as well as the organs associated with it, and the meridians that are interconnected with it.

**Notes for Acupuncturists**
This book is not intended as a study guide for acupuncturists. It does not include the Chinese name for the points, the needle insertion depth, or the angle of insertion. The points are listed by number only, except for points that do not have a commonly used number, such as the extra points. The meridians are listed in alphabetical order, to make the points easier to find.

In this book there is a difference between Liver and liver. The capitalized word refers to the Chinese theory of the liver. In some cases, the theories merge, but I have attempted to capitalize the organ if the function is different from the Western function.

# Chapter 1

## How Acupuncture Works

It is not necessary for you to understand how acupuncture works to treat yourself with acupressure, or to learn what each point does, but the beauty of Chinese medicine is that it has its own system of diagnosis and treatment. For example, it is not necessary to know exactly what type of digestive problem you have, the points that regulate your digestion can be treated, and your body heals itself.

### How Acupuncture Treats Pain

Pain is a large subject. There are so many ways that acupuncture can be used to relieve pain. The key thing to remember is that acupuncture of all types *restores normal blood flow to the area that hurts*. Pain is caused by a lack of healthy blood flow. After blood circulation is improved, the body can heal itself.

There are many options to treat pain. There are dozens of ways to treat each type of pain. Acupuncture also helps to break down scar tissue, and relax tight muscles. Nerve pain is relieved when acupuncture restores healthy circulation in the affected area.

When you get acupuncture to treat pain, in most cases other health issues can be treated at the same time. It is a truly holistic treatment. The whole body is treated. Acupuncture does not treat symptoms, it treats the underlying cause of the disease, and helps the body to completely resolve it.

## Local or Distal?

*Local* points are located near the site of pain. *Distal* points are located further away. Back pain can be treated by choosing from about 100 acupuncture points. There are points on the hand, arm, leg, ear, and other places that relieve back pain. The type of pain you have determines which points will be most effective. There are several points on the hand that are very strong to relieve back pain. The style of your acupuncturist also determines which points are chosen.

To treat pain, acupuncturists determine which meridian is affected. When points on the affected meridian are stimulated, it restores normal circulation. We also treat not only the affected meridian, but points on the stronger meridians in the area. Distal acupuncture is done by treating points that balance the affected meridian. There are hundreds of ways to treat pain with acupuncture. For example, a basic treatment for arm pain might include Large Intestine 4, 11, and 15. These points strongly restore healthy circulation in the arm.

## How Acupuncture Treats Emotions

In Chinese medicine, physical imbalances can lead to emotional imbalances. There is no separation of the mind and body. The mind affects the body, and vice versa. Treating the body with acupuncture and Chinese herbs is very beneficial to emotional health. You cannot be emotionally healthy if you are not physically healthy.

Emotions such as anxiety or stress are correlated to specific organ imbalances. Stress, for example, is related to your Liver. Anxiety is usually related to your Heart. Stress can be treated via the Liver meridian. Liver 2 and 3 are the most commonly used points for the Liver, although Spleen 6 also regulates the Liver. Anxiety and insomnia can be treated by regulating, and calming the Heart.

Points such as Pericardium 6, and Heart 7 are commonly used for anxiety and insomnia. There are often other imbalances that need to be treated. In fact, most people have multiple organ systems out of balance.

**Chinese Medicine Diagnosis**
A Chinese medicine diagnosis includes asking numerous questions. These questions tell us how your body is working. The questions might not seem to be related to your ailment, but they are in Chinese medicine. We will look at your tongue to see the general color and coating, as well as the shape. We take your pulse, which gives us more information about your health.

There are dozens of what we call *Organ Patterns* in Chinese medicine. You can have one, or you can have many of them. After a diagnosis has been made, acupuncture works to treat the underlying imbalances. Symptoms that seem to be unrelated to your health issue, can be very important in making your Chinese medicine diagnosis. The symptoms go away when the underlying imbalance is resolved.

## Yin and Yang

You might have heard about Yin and Yang and wondered what they were. The theory behind them is pretty extensive, but I want you to have a basic idea of what they are, because certain acupuncture points treat the Yin, and some treat the Yang.

Think of Yang as hot, dry, and energy. It is related to the drive, and testosterone can be associated with it. As we age, our Kidneys decline. That causes a reduction in hormones. Yin is the cool, and moist. Yin correlates to estrogen. We all have Yin and Yang. Men have more Yang than women do. Children have the most Yang. They are bundles of energy. That is a very basic explanation, but I want things to be easy to understand.

Yin and Yang must be sufficient for the body to be healthy. There are many herbal tonics that are used in Chinese medicine to strengthen the Yin and Yang of the kidneys to improve health as you age.

Although there are dozens of organ patterns, I want to explain the most common ones. The organ patterns in this section are the most commonly seen in clinic. If you understand how the organs function in Chinese medicine, it makes more sense how acupuncture can treat so many types of diseases.

Please remember that only *one* symptom is necessary to indicate that organ pattern is relevant for a health issue. In many cases, that is all someone will have, one symptom.

**Kidney Organ Patterns**

The most common imbalances in the Kidneys are a Yin or Yang deficiency. The kidneys are very important and treating the kidneys will resolve issues associated with aging. There are also anti-aging Chinese tonic herbs, which will improve energy levels, and treat disorders related to the Kidneys.

**Kidney Yang Deficiency**

Common symptoms of Kidney Yang deficiency include lower back pain, weak or painful knees, weak legs, feeling cold when others are comfortable, impotence, premature ejaculation, fatigue, frequent or profuse urination, apathy, swelling in the legs, and fertility problems. A Kidney Yang deficiency can often be correlated to a testosterone deficiency. In Chinese medicine theory, aging is associated with declining kidney energy. Ailments such as incontinence can often be resolved with acupuncture, and Chinese herbs.

**Kidney Yin Deficiency**

Common symptoms of a Kidney Yin deficiency are dizziness, tinnitus, poor memory, hearing issues or deafness, dry mouth at night, thirst, lower back pain, bone aches, insomnia, and night sweats. A Kidney Yin deficiency can often be correlated to an estrogen deficiency.

To treat Kidney imbalances, Kidney 3, 6, or 7 can be used. I like to combine all three points. Chinese herbs are often an important part of recovery from Kidney imbalances. Cordyceps is an example of a kidney tonic herb.

## Spleen and Stomach Organ Patterns

The Spleen in Chinese medicine theory is completely different from the function in Western medicine. The Spleen in Chinese medicine is associated with digestion and energy production. The most common imbalance is Spleen Qi deficiency.

## Spleen Qi Deficiency

A weak Spleen can cause a lack of appetite, abdominal bloating after eating, fatigue, pale complexion, weak arms and legs, loose stools. A spleen weakness can also cause excess fluid to be retained in the body. Stomach 36 is the strongest point to strengthen and regulate digestion, as well as improve energy levels. Weak digestion makes it more difficult to be completely healthy, as you do not get adequate nourishment from your food.

## Stomach Fire

Stomach fire symptoms include a burning pain in the stomach area, thirst for cold drinks, constant hunger, bleeding gums, acid reflux, constipation, vomiting after eating, and bad breath. This pattern is not common, but it is similar to gastritis, which is an inflammation of the stomach.

## Heart Organ Patterns

The Heart is affected by all emotions. Heart imbalances often cause anxiety, and insomnia. The Heart meridian is commonly used to treat Heart imbalances. Heart 5, 6, and 7 are often combined with Kidney points to treat the root imbalance. Stomach 36 can be used to improve energy levels, which impact the Heart.

## Heart Qi Deficiency

When the energy of the Heart is weak, it can cause heart palpitations, shortness of breath on exertion, unusual sweating, pale face, and fatigue. Palpitations are when you feel your heart beating.

## Heart Blood Deficiency

A deficiency of Heart blood can cause heart palpitations, dizziness, insomnia, poor memory, anxiety, being easily startled, a pale face and lips.

## Heart Yin Deficiency

A Heart Yin deficiency can cause heart palpitations, insomnia, being easily startled, poor memory, anxiety, feeling emotionally restless, flushed face, feeling of heat in the evening, night sweats, dry mouth and throat, and five palm heat, which is when the palms of your hands and feet feel hot. This pattern is common in menopause.

## Heart Fire

Heart fire causes heart palpitations, thirst, tongue ulcers, feeling agitated or restless, feeling hot, insomnia, facial redness, and a bitter taste in the mouth.

## Lung Organ Patterns

The Lungs can be treated with acupuncture to resolve colds and flu, treat asthma, bronchitis, and any ailment associated with the lungs. Strong lungs ensure healthy energy levels.

## Lung Qi Deficiency

A Lung Qi deficiency means the lung function is weak, which can cause shortness of breath, coughing, a weak voice, and a dislike of speaking. This can also be a side effect of a cold or flu. The coughing during a cold weakens the Lungs, which can cause a chronic weak cough. Some people never fully recover from a cold or flu, or bronchitis. The lungs remain weak. Herbs like cordyceps strengthen the lung energy, to help restore healthy lung function.

## Phlegm Heat Obstructing the Lungs

Excess mucus in the lungs can cause a barking cough, which is a deep cough that sounds like a dog barking, profuse yellow mucus, shortness of breath, asthma, and a stuffy feeling in your chest. This correlates to bronchitis in some cases. The type of cough tells you what is causing it. A light cough is from weak lungs, a deep and barking cough is when there is too much mucus and inflammation in the lungs.

Wheezing is a common symptom of phlegm heat in the lungs. The lungs can be strengthened by herbs like Reishi mushroom, and cordyceps. Red Reishi mushroom is also a longevity tonic. Always take wheezing seriously, it can indicate a bacterial infection in the lungs, which should be treated urgently.

After you see your medical doctor for wheezing, your acupuncturist can help. There are herbal formulas that help to resolve the mucus, strengthen the lungs, and stop the wheezing. Stomach 40 is called the *Phlegm Point*, and it helps resolve mucus, and Lung 5 clears heat, or inflammation, in the lungs.

Herbs like Andrographis are used in Chinese medicine to treat bacterial infections. There is a famous herbal formula called *Chuan Xin Lian* that is very effective for infections. Chinese herbs must be taken very often, sometimes every two to three hours, but in my experience, infections can be resolved in a few days. I think Chinese herbs will more popular over time, as antibiotics have been overused and there are many strains of drug resistant bacteria. The herbs are broad spectrum, and typically have no side effects. I always refer patients to a medical doctor to treat infections. Infections can be life threatening.

**Liver Organ Patterns**
The Liver in Chinese medicine theory is very different from the modern medicine theory. The Liver is strongly affected by stress. Regular stress stagnates the Liver energy, which causes many ailments. Most people have some degree of Liver stagnation. Liver 2 treats Liver fire, Liver 3 treats most other Liver patterns. Acupuncture and Chinese herbal medicine are very effective to relieve stress. They help to relieve the accumulation of a lifetime of stress. Migraine headaches are often caused by Liver imbalances.

**Liver Qi Stagnation**
Liver Qi stagnation causes feeling irritated or stressed, sighing, hiccup, depression, nausea, vomiting, acid reflux, belching, difficulty swallowing, irregular periods, painful periods, breast distention, and lumps in the breast or under the arms.

One of the more interesting symptoms of Liver Qi stagnation is sighing. You will sometimes notice that someone is sighing a lot. That is the Liver trying to relieve stagnation.

A Chinese herbal formula called *Xiao Yao San*, or *Free and Easy Wanderer*, is very popular to treat stress. This formula is available over the counter, and it is one of the most balanced herbal formulas, which means most people can take it. If everyone took this formula, there would be a lot less stress and depression in the world. Stress affects your liver, which becomes imbalanced and that can lead to depression. It is also a common cause of infertility.

## Liver Fire
Liver fire causes severe irritability, sudden outbursts of anger, tinnitus, headaches on the side of the head, dizziness, thirst, bitter taste, and a sudden flushed feeling when angry. Liver fire also causes facial sweating. When under stress, the heat flares up to the face, making it feel hot. Liver 2 is the best point for Liver fire.

## Liver Blood Deficiency
Liver blood deficiency symptoms include blurred vision, floaters in the eyes, dizziness, insomnia, lack of menstruation, muscle cramps, brittle nails, and muscle weakness.

In Chinese medicine a blood deficiency is what causes eye floaters. If you have floaters, you can see black spots floating in front of your eyes if you look at a white wall. Many people have these and do not know it. They also rarely believe me when I tell them it can be fixed. It takes about a month. Blood tonic herbs need to be taken to restore healthy blood. I always have patients see an eye doctor to ensure there is no physical eye problem. A detached retina can also cause floaters.

Muscle cramps are also commonly seen with a blood deficiency. If there is not enough blood to keep the muscles nourished, they become tight and can cramp up. This can also cause neck and shoulder pain, as well as migraines.

Liver Fire is treated with Liver 2, and 3. A Liver blood deficiency would need to be treated by herbs, as well as points like Stomach 36 to improve energy production, and Spleen 6 to nourish the blood. Liver issues often cause menstrual problems, and infertility.

**Dampness and Phlegm**
It is a little difficult to explain the concept of dampness and phlegm in a short space. In Chinese medicine when the body accumulates too much fluid it is called dampness, which is called edema in Western medicine. In Chinese medicine theory dampness can be caused by either a weak Spleen, or weak Kidneys failing to remove the excess fluids. Chinese medicine is very effective to treat edema, it treats the root of the disorder by strengthening the organs responsible for fluid transportation in the body.

Phlegm is how Chinese medicine describes mucus. The mucus can be in your lungs during a cold or flu, and other ailments such as bronchitis. There is another type of phlegm that is not something you would see during a cold or flu. The word "phlegm" describes swellings in the body and imbalances that block organ function. Stomach 40 is the *Phlegm Point*. It treats all types of phlegm. Stomach 36 would also be included in your treatment, this point has dozens of functions.

These organ patterns are just the most commonly seen organ patterns in the clinic. This information is from Giovanni Maciocia's book *The Foundations of Chinese Medicine*. This is the textbook acupuncture students use their first year in school. It is an amazing book. If you would like to study Chinese medicine, I strongly recommend this book. There is no other book that really explains Chinese medicine like this book does. I am only giving a quick overview of common ailments, so the acupuncture points make more sense to you. Now, when your acupuncturist tells you that you have Liver fire, or Liver Qi stagnation, you will understand what he or she is talking about.

# Chapter 2

## How to Locate Acupuncture Points

Acupuncture points are located by using anatomical landmarks. For example, Pericardium 6 is located 2 cun from the wrist crease. You measure 2 cun by using your fingers. If you are treating someone who has smaller or larger fingers, you will use their measurements to locate the points. That means you would use their thumb size, rather than your own. You can also measure the point, and adjust the location slightly according to their measurements.

Many points are located using bony landmarks as a reference. The medial malleolus is an example of this. This is the round bone on the inside of the ankle. You place your fingers over the tip of the medial malleolus to locate the Kidney meridian points.

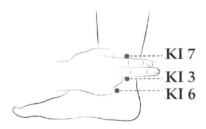

Kidney 3 is at the same level as the tip of the medial malleolus bone. Kidney 7 is 2 cun above Kidney 3, and Kidney 6 is below the medial malleolus.

## Point Diameter

The size of each acupuncture point can be large. As long as you are inside the area, the point will be activated. The diameter can be the size of a nickel or quarter.

## Cun Measurement

To locate acupuncture points, you need to have a way to measure distances on the body. That measurement unit is called a *cun*. That is the Chinese word for it. It is pronounced "Soon." Each cun is the size of your thumb knuckle. You will need to measure 1 cun, 1.5 cun, 2 cun, 3 cun, and 4 cun. If you are in doubt, you can always default to your thumb to do the measurement.

1 cun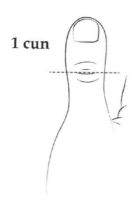

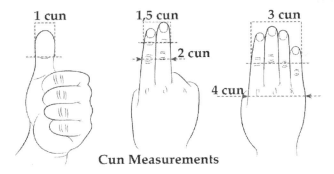

Cun Measurements

## Anatomy Terms

The point locations in this book are explained as simply as possible. In some cases, I have used anatomy terms that might not be familiar to you. Rest assured that the images make the points easy to locate. The anatomy terms are used, but in most cases you can simply look at the image.

A few terms that you will see often include:

## Medial Malleolus

This is the round bone on the inside of your ankle. This bone is used to locate points in the area, such as Kidney 3, 6, and 7, as well as Spleen 6.

## Lateral Malleolus

This is the round bone on the outside of your ankle. This bone is used to locate points on the Bladder and Gallbladder meridians. It is also used as a point of measurement to find other points on the leg, such as Stomach 40.

**Border of the Red and White Skin**
This is a term that explains where the skin changes color. It is usually at the border of the sole of your foot, or the palm of your hand. It is not necessary to be able to see this to find the points to do acupressure.

# Chapter 3

## How to Do Acupressure Effectively

In order for acupressure to work, the point needs to be activated. With acupuncture, a needle is inserted into the point, which stimulates circulation in the point, which activates it. Acupuncture needles are tiny, about the size of a hair.

To activate the points using acupressure, there are several options.

- Pressing firmly with your fingers
- Using magnetic pellets on a piece of tape, which are applied to the acupuncture points and left on for a specific period of time, such as eight hours
- Using tiny seeds on a piece of tape that is applied to the ear. The seeds can be vaccaria seeds or other types of pellets such as ionic beads, or magnetic pellets
- Mini massager

The important thing to remember is that you must press firmly enough to activate the point. When you get acupuncture, the needles stay in place for about 30 minutes. While you relax, the needles have time to do their job. When doing acupressure, you will need to press firmly enough and long enough to stimulate the point. I would say five minutes per point is usually enough, but in some cases

10 minutes is necessary. It depends on which point is being treated, and how sick you are.

**Treatment Frequency**

Acupressure, like acupuncture, is a form of therapy. It is most effective if done daily. Every time you do acupuncture or acupressure, you are stimulating the body to function normally. If you only do it once a week, it will be less effective. Acupuncture and acupressure are both types of therapy, which means you need to do a *series* of treatments to get better.

Please do not expect one treatment of any sort to be all you need. I would plan on doing a series of four to eight treatments, and then decide if you need to continue. It can also be used for occasional problems such as nausea. The best point for nausea is Pericardium 6, which also treats insomnia.

**Mini Massagers**

Mini massagers are about 4 inches long, and they are used by some people for things other than acupressure. They are the perfect size to do acupressure. You can easily take them with you, and the tip is about half an inch in diameter, which makes it perfect to treat an acupuncture point. The best massagers for acupressure come with several different types of heads. The ones with the larger number of prongs seem to be the most effective for acupressure. These massagers cost about $10, and they can be bought online.

These massagers are also marketed to be used for scar treatments. Improving blood flow to a scar helps the body to break it down. Acupuncture is amazing to treat scars, as well as non-healing wounds, that are common in diabetics. Placing the needles around the wound improves blood flow, which helps the body to close the wound. A lack of healing is caused by a lack of circulation.

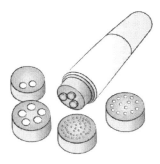

**Magnetic Pellets**

Magnetic pellets provide very strong stimulation to the points. I use the Helio brand of pellets, they come in a box of 100 pellets and each magnet is 800 gauss. Gauss is a measurement of how strong a magnet is. I have found these pellets to be very effective for insomnia, when placed on Pericardium 6. It is best to limit the time magnets are left on the body to eight hours. You might not feel them working, but they are very strong.

**Acupressure Duration**

The effects of acupressure are not usually felt immediately. It usually takes about an hour, although it depends on which point is being treated, and what results you are expecting. If you are doing acupressure on points like Large Intestine 11, to treat constipation, or Pericardium 6 to treat insomnia, you will usually see results in about an hour. If you do not see results, you can do acupressure again.

**Getting the Qi**
When you stimulate an acupuncture point, you are activating the point. Once the point has been activated, it starts to work. Acupuncturists call that "Getting the Qi," which is necessary for acupuncture or acupressure to work. The signs that you have activated a point include the following sensations in the area being treated:

- Itching
- Tingling
- Numbness
- Aching (more common in strong points like Stomach 36)
- Warmth

Sometimes you cannot describe how it feels, you just know something is going on, you feel the increase in blood flow. Even if you do not feel anything that does not mean that nothing is happening. If you have very low energy levels, you will be less likely to feel anything until your energy levels are built up, which usually takes about a month.

**Ear Acupressure**
Ear acupressure is another way to treat yourself. The ear is very sensitive to any type of stimulation. You can buy ear seeds online. There are several different types. The seeds are placed on a tiny square piece of tape. After applying the seeds to the ear, the tape will last a couple of days,

depending on how often you shampoo, and how strong the tape is.

I like Sakamura ion pellets. They come in two types, the tape is either clear or flesh colored, and the pellets are either gold or silver. It is a matter of personal preference. I use clear tape with gold pellets. It is best to remove the pellets after two days and switch to the other ear.

# Chapter 4

## Ear Acupuncture or Acupressure

The ear is a microcosm of the whole body. That means the whole body is represented on the ear. The map of the ear shows the body represented as an upside down fetus. All ailments can be treated on the ear. The ear can be used to treat internal organ imbalances, pain, emotional issues, and to regulate the entire body.

The image below shows the inverted fetus. You will notice the head at the bottom of the image. The internal organs are located on the inner part of the ear, by the ear canal.

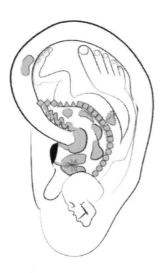

Some acupuncturists specialize in ear acupuncture. Many acupuncturists combine ear acupuncture with body acupuncture to get the benefits of both. Ear acupuncture and acupressure are especially useful to treat pain. Just locate the area on the ear that corresponds to the body part that is painful.

The ear points can be stimulated using tiny acupuncture needles, ear seeds that are made with vaccaria seeds, which are tiny black seeds that are placed on a small piece of tape. The seeds are placed on the ear and can be left on several days, they usually fall off within a few days. It is common to alternate ears, which means that for one treatment the right ear is treated, and the left ear is treated for the following visit.

**Ear Seeds**
The image below shows vaccaria seeds on little plastic flats, you just unpeel the piece of tape and place it on the ear. Using tweezers makes it easier.

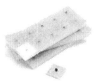

There are numerous types of small pellets typically used on the ear. Another type of ear pellet is Magrain Ion pellets from Sakamura. These are tiny beads, either gold or silver, attached to round pieces of tape. The beads are treated to provide stimulation that is not as strong as a magnet, but stronger than a vaccaria seed.

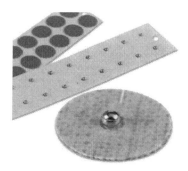

This image shows Sakamura Magrain Ion pellets on flesh colored tape. There are two options, clear tape, or flesh colored tape, and gold or silver pellets. Your acupuncturist will have a personal preference on which type of pellets are used.

Ear acupuncture is also used to help relieve drug addiction. Ear acupuncture relieves stress and can be used by non-acupuncturists to help in addiction protocols. The following image shows the NADA ear protocol used by addiction specialists. NADA stands for National Acupuncture Detoxification Association. There is special training offered for those interested in learning the protocol. For more information, please refer to www.acudetox.com.

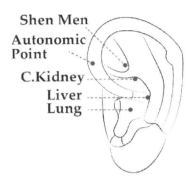

The following chart shows the spine represented on the ear. The points C1 to C7 represent the cervical, or neck vertebrae. I have found that treating these points on the ear with Sakamura pellets is as effective as any other type of neck treatment. Just place the pellets on the edge of the ear in the corresponding affected area and press firmly. When you press firmly, it will hurt a little. It will only hurt if there is a problem in that area. The points T1 to T 12 treat the thoracic, or upper back area. L1 to L5 are for the lumbar, or lower back area. S1 and 2 are for the sacrum, or tailbone.

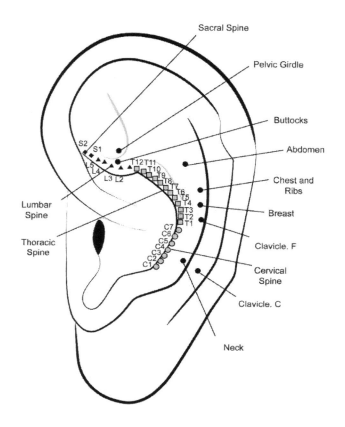

## Commonly Used Ear Points

### Shen Men
Shen Men is a master point. It calms the mind, relieves stress, pain, anxiety, insomnia, and it is used in combination with other points. The name means "Spirit Gate." It is one of the most commonly used points on the ear.

### Point Zero
This point balances the body. It helps to regulate hormones, and calm the brain.

### Tranquilizer Point
This point is also called the Relaxation Point, or Valium Analogue Point, by Terry Oleson. It is sedating, and relaxing and can be used to treat anxiety, high blood pressure, and chronic stress.

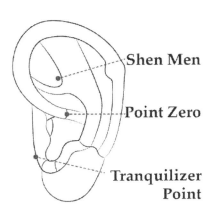

Shen Men

Point Zero

Tranquilizer
Point

There are several systems of ear acupuncture. If you interested in further study, the book *Auriculotherapy Manual* by Terry Oleson, PhD, is a good choice.

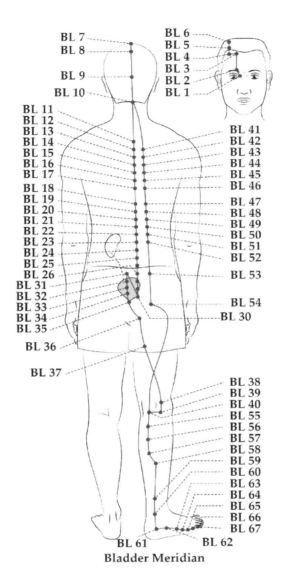

BL 7
BL 8
BL 9
BL 10
BL 11
BL 12
BL 13
BL 14
BL 15
BL 16
BL 17
BL 18
BL 19
BL 20
BL 21
BL 22
BL 23
BL 24
BL 25
BL 26
BL 31
BL 32
BL 33
BL 34
BL 35
BL 36
BL 37

BL 6
BL 5
BL 4
BL 3
BL 2
BL 1

BL 41
BL 42
BL 43
BL 44
BL 45
BL 46
BL 47
BL 48
BL 49
BL 50
BL 51
BL 52
BL 53
BL 54
BL 30

BL 38
BL 39
BL 40
BL 55
BL 56
BL 57
BL 58
BL 59
BL 60
BL 63
BL 64
BL 65
BL 66
BL 67

BL 61
BL 62

Bladder Meridian

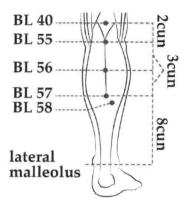

## Bladder 40

Located at the midpoint of the popliteal fossa. Translation: located behind the knee, at roughly the midpoint.

## Functions and Common Usage

Strengthens the lower back to relieve back pain. It relaxes the tendons, and can be used to treat back pain that causes stiffness, and the inability to stand up straight.

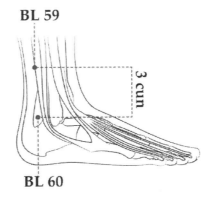

## Bladder 60
In the depression between the lateral malleolus and the calcaneal tendon. Translation: located between the ankle bone on the outside of the ankle, and the tendon on the back of the heel.

## Functions and Common Usage
- Ankle pain
- Childhood convulsions
- Headaches on the back of the head, occipital headaches
- Heel pain
- Labor induction, should not be used during pregnancy
- Lower back pain
- Lower leg paralysis
- Neck pain
- Pain in the sole of the foot
- Regulates the Bladder meridian to relieve pain on the meridian
- Relaxes the tendons

- Sacrum pain
- Sciatica
- Seizures
- Severe, sudden back pain that makes walking difficult
- Vertigo

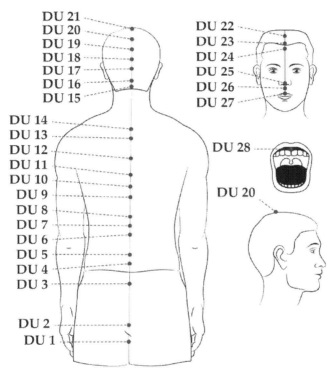

DU 21
DU 20
DU 19
DU 18
DU 17
DU 16
DU 15
DU 14
DU 13
DU 12
DU 11
DU 10
DU 9
DU 8
DU 7
DU 6
DU 5
DU 4
DU 3
DU 2
DU 1

DU 22
DU 23
DU 24
DU 25
DU 26
DU 27
DU 28
DU 20

**Du Meridian - Governing Vessel**

The Du meridian is the Chinese name for the meridian that runs along the spine. It is also called the Governing vessel. It is most commonly referred to by the Chinese name, so that is what I will use here.

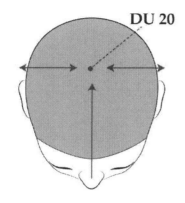

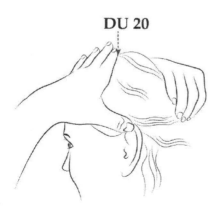

**How to Locate Du 20**

**Du 20**

Located 7 cun above the posterior hairline. You can use your hands to locate this point. Place the tip of your thumbs at the top of your ears, and your fingertips will meet at the top of your head at the approximate location of Du 20. You will feel a slight indentation at the point.

**Functions and Common Usage**
- Benefits the head and brain
- Calms the mind
- Improves concentration
- Improves memory
- Insomnia
- Opens the sinuses to treat sinus blockage
- Prolapse of the uterus or rectum
- Raises energy and descends it as needed, it regulates circulation
- Restores collapsed Yang
- Revives consciousness

This point can be used to treat prolapse of the rectum, as well as uterine prolapse. It improves memory by increasing blood flow to the brain. It opens the sinuses to treat nasal obstructions that can cause sinus headaches. Collapsed Yang is when the body is so weak that the person faints or passes out.

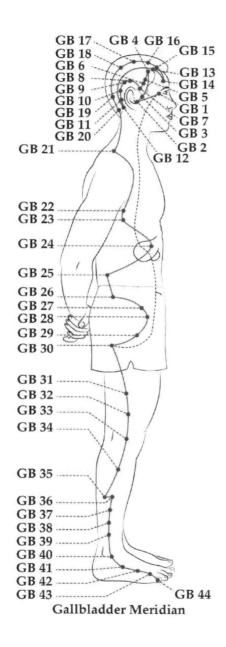

GB 17   GB 4   GB 16
GB 18                    GB 15
GB 6
GB 8                     GB 13
GB 9                     GB 14
GB 10                    GB 5
GB 19                    GB 1
GB 11                    GB 7
GB 20                    GB 3
GB 21                    GB 2
                   GB 12

GB 22
GB 23

GB 24

GB 25

GB 26
GB 27
GB 28
GB 29
GB 30

GB 31
GB 32
GB 33
GB 34

GB 35

GB 36
GB 37
GB 38
GB 39
GB 40
GB 41
GB 42
GB 43                    GB 44

**Gallbladder Meridian**

As you can see from the meridian image, this meridian wraps around the side of the head three times. Many of the points on the side of the head are not commonly used. It is hard to describe the location of these points without using anatomy terms. I will highlight, and bullet point the most commonly used points, as usual. Migraine headaches often affect the Gallbladder meridian. It is not common to use the points on the head for migraines. Points on the Liver and Gallbladder meridians on the feet are often used to relieve migraines.

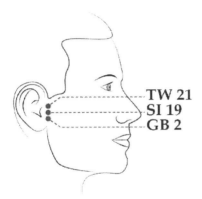

TW 21
SI 19
GB 2

**Gallbladder 2**
Anterior to the intertragic notch, on the posterior border of the condyloid process of the mandible. Locate with the mouth open. Translation: located in front of the ear. Please see the image for this one.

**Functions and Common Usage**
Opens the ears to treat deafness, tinnitus, ear infections and discharge, as well as ear pain. Treats hearing loss, jaw pain, and TMJ pain.

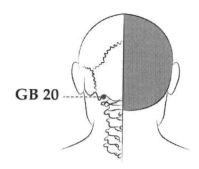

GB 20

## Gallbladder 20

In the hollow between the sternocleidomastoid and trapezius muscles.

## Functions and Common Usage

- Blurred vision
- Cold and flu
- Dizziness
- Gallbladder meridian pain
- Headaches
- Improves circulation to the eyes
- Loss of speech after a stroke
- Migraines
- Neck pain and stiffness
- Opens blocked ears
- Shoulder pain

## Clinical Notes

Gallbladder 20 is very strong to restore normal circulation in the head and neck. It can be used in combination with other points to treat migraine headaches. Most migraines are caused by tight muscles, or blockages in a meridian.

The Gallbladder meridian is very commonly affected. Migraines can also be treated by using other points at the opposite end of the Gallbladder meridian, as well as by restoring normal circulation to any area that has a blockage.

Stress causes tight muscles, which then reduce normal blood flow to the brain. Where there is a lack of healthy blood flow, there is pain. It also treats dizziness, which can be caused by tight muscles compressing nerves that affect the ear function.

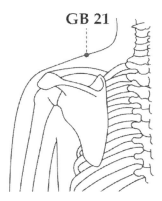

GB 21

## Gallbladder 21
Located halfway between the spine and the tip of the acromion bone.

## Functions and Common Usage
- Relieves pain in the neck and shoulders
- Treats breast pain, and breast abscess
- Insufficient lactation
- Should not be used during pregnancy, because it could induce labor

This point is often combined with GB 20 to treat neck pain, because it releases the tight muscles that cause neck and shoulder pain.

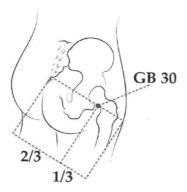

## Gallbladder 30

On the back side of the hip joint, one third of the way from the greater trochanter, which is the head of the thigh bone, and the top of the sacrum.

### Functions and Common Usage

- Buttock pain
- Hemiplegia
- Hip pain
- Leg atrophy
- Lower back pain
- Sciatica

### Clinical Notes

Gallbladder 30 is very effective to treat hip pain, and sciatica. The Gallbladder meridian runs down the side of the leg, to the foot. Sciatica often travels this exact course.

It sometimes stops at the knee, but if it is not treated, the sciatic pain can radiate all the way to the foot. Lower back issues must also be considered as a potential factor in hip pain. Herniated discs or tight muscles can easily affect the hip.

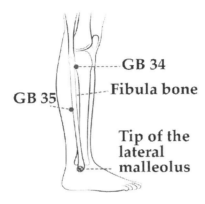

## Gallbladder 34
In the depression in front of and below the head of the fibula bone.

### Functions and Common Usage
- Calf muscle atrophy
- Contraction of foot tendons
- Hemiplegia
- Hypertension associated with the Liver imbalances
- Knee pain
- Regulates the liver and gallbladder
- Relaxes the tendons to relieve muscle spasms
- Rib pain
- Sciatica

## Clinical Notes

This point is used to treat any problem with tendons. It is also used to treat stress, because it treats the Liver, which is associated with stress in Chinese medicine.

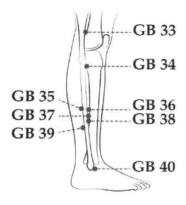

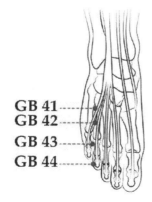

## Gallbladder 41

Located in the depression between the fourth and fifth metatarsal bones, on the lateral side of the extensor tendon. Translation: Between the fourth and fifth bones of the foot.

**Functions and Common Usage**

- Foot pain
- Headaches
- Migraine headaches
- Pain on the occiput (base of the skull)
- Regulates the Liver
- Spastic pain of the feet, or toes
- Toe pain

This point can be used to treat many types of headaches, as well as it is listed as facilitating lactation in one source.

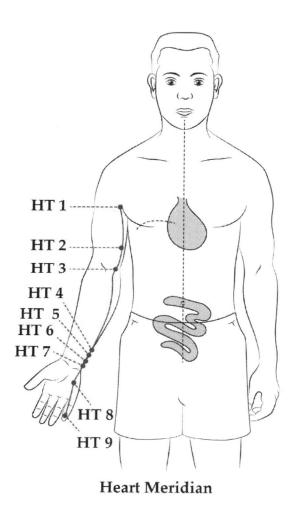

**Heart Meridian**

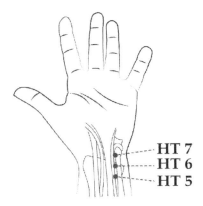

HT 7
HT 6
HT 5

## Heart 5

Located 1 cun above the wrist crease, on the radial side of the flexor carpi tendon.

### Functions and Common Usage
- Calms the mind
- Heart Fire
- Heart pounding sensation
- Palpitations (when you feel your heart beating)
- Regulates the Heart rhythm
- Strengthens the Heart
- Stuttering
- Sudden loss of voice with tongue stiffness

Heart 5 regulates the heart rhythm, which can treat heart arrhythmia. Acupressure is very effective on this point. Press your fingernail deeply into the point and hold for at least 5 minutes. Regular treatment will regulate and strengthen the heart.

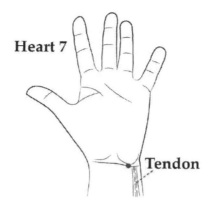

## Heart 7

Located at the wrist crease, on the radial side of the flexor carpi ulnaris tendon. There might be two wrist creases, and some people have three. This point is located at the level of the largest wrist crease.

## Functions and Common Usage

- Anxiety
- Calms the mind
- Heart arrhythmia
- Heart palpitations (you feel your heart beating)
- Heart pounding sensation
- Insomnia
- Irritability
- Manic depression
- Memory
- Regulates and strengthens the Heart

Heart 7 is one of the most important points on the body. It is a top point to treat anxiety and insomnia. It is a very calming point. Acupressure is effective on this point, you can either use your fingernail on this point, or use a magnetic pellet. It treats disorders caused by Heart imbalances, such as poor memory, irritability, and mania.

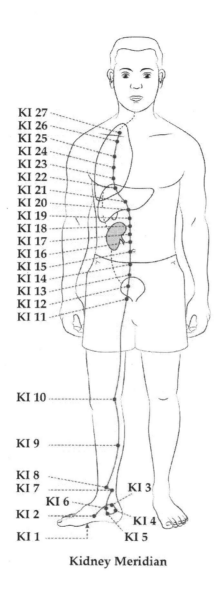

KI 27
KI 26
KI 25
KI 24
KI 23
KI 22
KI 21
KI 20
KI 19
KI 18
KI 17
KI 16
KI 15
KI 14
KI 13
KI 12
KI 11

KI 10

KI 9

KI 8
KI 7
KI 6
KI 2
KI 1

KI 3
KI 4
KI 5

**Kidney Meridian**

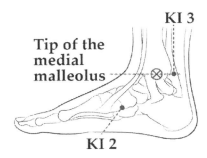

**Kidney 3**
In the depression between the medial malleolus, which is the ankle bone, and the back of the leg. Locate the point halfway between the tip of the medial malleolus and the back of the leg.

**Functions and Common Usage**
- Asthma
- Deafness
- Fatigue from Kidney weakness
- Frequent urination
- Heel pain
- Incontinence
- Insomnia
- Memory issues
- Strengthens Kidney Yang, which is associated with urination issues
- Strengthens the lower back and knees, helps to relieve back pain and knee weakness
- Strongly strengthens the kidneys
- Tinnitus
- Urgent urination

- Wheezing

Kidney 3 is the most important point on the Kidney meridian. It is used to treat any type of kidney issue, including frequent or urgent urination, incontinence, waking at night to urinate, and it calms the fetus. It can be used to treat ear disorders like deafness, tinnitus, as well as kidney stones. It can also treat insomnia that is caused by a kidney weakness.

## Clinical Notes

In Chinese medicine, the kidneys are the root of health. If you can keep your kidneys strong and healthy, you will live longer and be healthier. The kidneys are also one of the most important things affecting your energy level. Fatigue can be caused by weak kidneys. I like to combine this point with Kidney 7 and Kidney 6 for a stronger effect.

I have used this three point combination, Kidney 3, 6, and 7, to treat a patient who was on kidney dialysis. After a few weeks of treatment, she no longer needed dialysis. These points strengthened her kidneys enough so they could function on their own. I would never make a claim that I can cure kidney disease with these points, but in her case she was able to discontinue her kidney dialysis, after having received that treatment for several years.

Kidney dialysis filters the blood. This is necessary when the kidneys are too weak to sufficiently filter the blood. If you strengthen the Kidneys with acupuncture, the function of the kidneys is improved. Acupressure would be helpful for this. Acupuncture is much stronger, but you can benefit the kidneys by using acupressure on Kidney 3, 6, and 7.

I also used Kidney 3, 6, and 7 on another patient who had kidney problems. She had been told that her kidney function was declining, probably due to a reaction to an antibiotic. Her medical doctor told her she might have to go on dialysis. With weekly acupuncture she had restored kidney health and did not have to go on dialysis.

Something to consider about the kidney points is the effect they have on the emotions. The kidneys are associated with drive and willpower. If your kidneys are weak, you will suffer from fatigue and your drive to get ahead will be reduced. For a severe kidney deficiency, Chinese herbs are very effective to quickly restore the emotional aspect of the kidneys. Weak kidneys can also cause you to feel cold in general, as well as cause hot flashes.

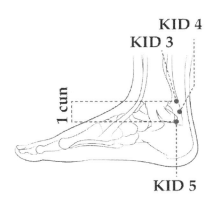

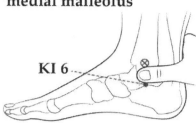

Tip of the
medial malleolus

KI 6

## Kidney 6

In the depression of the lower border of the medial malleolus, 1 cun below the medial malleolus, or inner ankle bone.

## Functions and Common Usage

- Asthma
- Calms the mind
- Constipation
- Dribbling urination
- Edema
- Expedites labor, do not use during pregnancy
- Frequent urination
- Hot flashes
- Insomnia
- Irregular menstruation
- Moistens the throat
- Sleeping too much
- Sore throat
- Strengthens the kidneys
- Uterine prolapse

Kidney 6 can be used for a sore or dry throat. It is a major point for insomnia, it is very calming. It also treats urinary issues such as frequent urination, and incontinence.

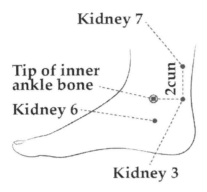

**Kidney 7**

Located 2 cun above Kidney 3.

**Functions and Common Usage**
- Dry mouth
- Edema, which is the abnormal retention of fluid causing swelling, often in the ankles and feet
- Foot pain
- Frequent urination due to Kidney weakness
- Incontinence
- Lower back pain
- Nephritis
- Night sweating
- Regulates sweating
- Regulates the bladder
- Regulates urination
- Strengthens the kidneys

Kidney 7 is a major point and it can be used to treat all aspects of the kidneys. It is especially useful to treat incontinence, although Chinese herbs are also very important for this. Edema is caused by your body not being able to get rid of fluid. You can test yourself by pressing firmly on your ankle for 30 seconds. If there is a depression remaining after you remove your finger, this is a sign that you are retaining fluid. It is very important to treat this. It is a sign that something is not functioning properly. Chinese medicine can treat the root cause of this problem.

Kidney 7 is especially used to treat urinary problems, which include painful urination, and nephritis.

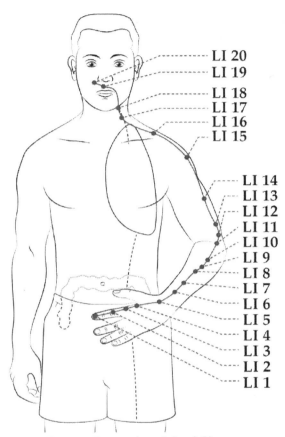

LI 20
LI 19
LI 18
LI 17
LI 16
LI 15
LI 14
LI 13
LI 12
LI 11
LI 10
LI 9
LI 8
LI 7
LI 6
LI 5
LI 4
LI 3
LI 2
LI 1

**Large Intestine Meridian**

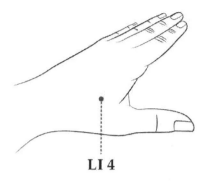

LI 4

## Large Intestine 4

Between the first and second metacarpal bones, in the middle of the second metacarpal bone, on the radial side.

## Functions and Common Usage

- Allergies
- Arm pain
- Cold and flu
- Constipation
- Deafness
- Ear infections
- Hand pain
- Headaches
- Hives
- Induces labor (it should not be used during pregnancy)
- Nosebleed
- Regulates sweating
- Regulates the face – can treat all face disorders

- Regulates the immune system
- Regulates the Lungs
- Sinus congestion
- Sore throat
- Toothache, lower jaw
- Treats the eyes, nose, mouth, and ears

This is one of the most commonly used points on the body. It is used to treat any issue on the head. It is often combined with Liver 3 to strongly relax the body and balance energy circulation, and relieve pain anywhere in the body. This treatment is called "Four Gates."

Large Intestine 4 is indispensable to treat allergies, and colds and flu. Combine it with Large Intestine 11, Stomach 36, and Stomach 40. Treat every two hours. It boosts the immune system so your body can clear viruses. It treats allergies by regulating and strengthening the immune system, so your body stops overreacting. This is the first choice for acupressure to treat headaches. Acupressure is very effective on this point.

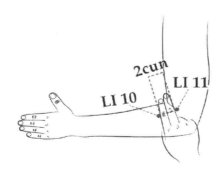

## Large Intestine 10

Located 2 cun from Large Intestine 11, on the line connecting LI 5 and LI 11.

## Functions and Common Usage

- Arm atrophy
- Arm pain
- Hemiplegia
- Indigestion
- Regulates the intestines
- Regulates the stomach
- Shoulder pain
- Toothache
- Treats arm paralysis after a stroke by strongly stimulating circulation in the Large Intestine meridian

Large Intestine 10 is commonly used to improve circulation in the arm. It can be combined with other points on the meridian such as LI 4, LI 11, and LI 15 to restore healthy blood flow in the arm. Combining points on a meridian is a common way to restore circulation. Using one point alone is often not enough to treat the problem. Strong stimulation of this point can send noticeable warmth to the hands, if they feel cold or the circulation is impaired.

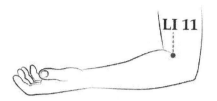

**Large Intestine 11**
Located halfway between the elbow crease and the elbow.
Locate with the arm bent, as shown in the image.

**Functions and Common Usage**
- Allergies
- Arm atrophy after a stroke, combine with LI 4, LI 10, and LI 15
- Arm numbness
- Arm pain
- Cold and flu
- Constipation – it regulates and moistens the large intestine
- Eczema
- Elbow pain
- Fever reduction
- Heatstroke
- Herpes zoster
- High blood pressure
- Hives
- Itching
- Pain on the Large Intestine meridian

- Psoriasis
- Rashes
- Regulates the Lungs
- Shoulder pain
- Shoulder stiffness
- Skin diseases of all types
- Sore throat
- Strengthens the immune system

## Clinical Notes

You can see from the length of this list that Large Intestine 11 is a major point. It clears heat due to many causes, so it treats skin disorders caused by heat, which means inflammatory skin disorders. It is combined with LI 4, ST 36, and ST 40 to resolve colds and flu. It is combined with LI 4 to treat allergies. It is combined with LI 4, SP 6, and LV 3 to treat food allergies. This point combination helps to balance the immune system so it stops overreacting to substances.

Once I had a patient who was very sick, but she refused to see a medical doctor. She was red and very hot, and was showing signs of delirium. I suspected she was dehydrated, and not able to be rational. I used Large Intestine 11 to quickly reduce her fever, and asked her husband to call an ambulance.

This point is very effective when treated with acupressure. I recommend using the thumb to press deeply enough. You will basically be pressing in at the end of the elbow crease.

Large Intestine 11 is the top point to use for constipation. It can be combined with Stomach 36 to regulate the intestines. You can press on both elbows at the same time, or alternate with five minutes on each one. I also use this point to treat patients who have had abdominal surgery. Large Intestine 11 regulates the intestines, which restores normal bowel function after surgery. Surgery disrupts normal intestinal function because the nerves are severed.

Large Intestine 11 is often used in combination with other points on the arm, such as LI 4, LI 10, and LI 15 to restore the function of the arm after a stroke, or after the arm is broken or injured.

This point can be used to treat intestinal problems in babies. It quickly relieves constipation, as well as irregularity of intestinal function. Babies respond quickly to acupressure.

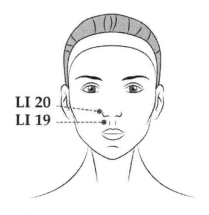

## Large Intestine 20
Located at the naso-labial groove, at the level of the midpoint of the lateral border of the nostril.

## Functions and Common Usage
- Loss of sense of smell
- Mouth deviation, which is when the mouth is crooked due to Bell's palsy or other nerve conditions
- Nasal polyps
- Nosebleeds
- Opens the sinuses
- Sinus headaches
- Trigeminal neuralgia

Large Intestine 20 will open the sinuses to relieve sinus pressure and headaches. It treats loss of sense of smell by opening the sinuses and restoring normal circulation. Mouth deviation and trigeminal neuralgia are treated by the effect this point has on the local nerves. As in all acupuncture, healthy nerve function and circulation are restored, which will treat numerous issues in the affected area.

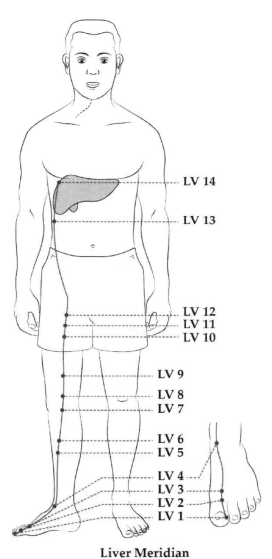

**Liver Meridian**

75

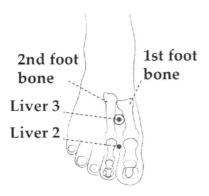

## Liver 2
Between the big toe and the second toe, in the web margin.

## Functions and Common Usage
- Abnormal uterine bleeding from Fire, which is extreme heat
- Clears Liver Fire
- Convulsions
- Dizziness
- Genital pain
- Headache
- Hepatitis
- Hernia
- Hypertension
- Insomnia
- Jaundice
- Menstrual problems including pain
- Nosebleed
- Regulates Liver Qi

- Seizures
- Severe irritability, with a sensation of heat in the face
- Stops bleeding due to heat syndromes
- Subdues Liver Yang
- Tinnitus
- Treats damp heat in the lower abdomen, this can manifest as many things, including a urinary tract infection
- Treats depression caused by Liver issues

Liver 2 is a major point, it treats symptoms of Liver Fire, and heat in the blood. Bear in mind that some of these symptoms can be caused by other imbalances. Tinnitus, for example, can be related to a Kidney weakness. A full diagnosis must be done for all symptoms.

Liver 2 is a top point for irritability. It strongly purges heat or Fire in the Liver and relieves stress. This point can be combined with Liver 3. It treats the emotions when someone is very irritable, gets a flushed face, or a hot sensation in the face when irritated or stressed. If a person "blows up" or is easily angered, consider using this point. Liver 2 and 3 are used to treat stress, which is caused most often by Liver imbalances in Chinese medicine.

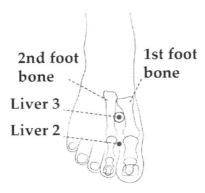

## Liver 3

Located between the first and second toes, about 1.5 cun above the web of the toe. Please note that the size of your feet bones determines how far this point is from the toe web, everyone is different. It is located in the depression between the first and second metatarsal bones (bones in the feet).

To locate Liver 3 you can run your finger from the toe web to the foot bones, you will find a small indentation right before you get to the bones of the feet. The image shows the point with a circle around it, so you can see that Liver 3 is located in a small hollow on the foot.

## Functions and Common Usage

- Blurred vision
- Dizziness
- Eye conditions
- Frequent sighing
- Headaches
- Hepatitis
- Hernia

- High blood pressure
- Insomnia
- Irregular menstruation
- Jaundice
- Migraine headaches
- Morning sickness
- Nausea
- Regulates blood
- Regulates hormones
- Regulates Liver Qi
- Relaxes the entire body
- Restless fetus disorder, acupuncture helps to calm the baby in utero
- Sedates Liver Yang rising
- Stress relief
- Treats depression caused by stress
- Uterine prolapse
- Vertigo, main point
- Vision problems
- Vomiting

Most people need to have Liver 3 treated. It relieves stress, and it is very relaxing. It treats all diseases that originate in the Liver as viewed by Chinese medicine. It treats migraine headaches and helps to relieve muscle tension. Acupressure is effective on this point. A magnetic pellet can be applied as needed. Remember to remove magnetic pellets after eight hours, or the point will stop responding to treatment temporarily.

Liver Yang rising is often seen in high blood pressure. The stress affects the Liver, which then rises to the head.

Controlling anger and high blood pressure are important to prevent strokes. Acupuncture relieves stress, and anger.

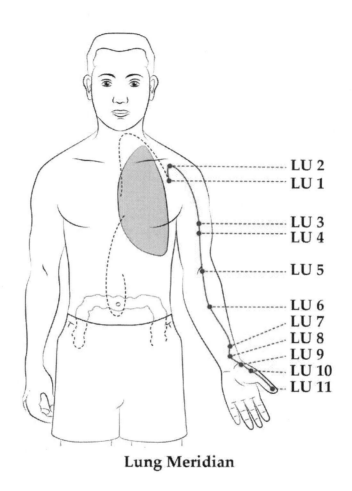

**Lung Meridian**

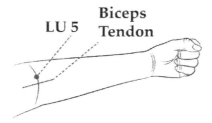

## Lung 5

On the elbow crease, on the thumb side of the biceps tendon. Locate the point with the elbow flexed. When you make a fist, the tendon becomes more prominent.

### Functions and Common Usage

- Bronchitis
- Clears heat from the Lungs
- Colds and flu
- Cough
- Inflammatory lung conditions
- Regulates the Lung function
- Shortness of breath
- Wheezing

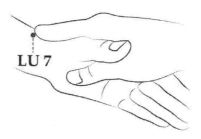

**Lung 7**
Above the styloid process of the radius bone, 1.5 cun above the wrist crease. Located in the depression between the two tendons above the wrist. To locate, place your hands together across each other as shown in the image.

**Functions and Common Usage**
- Bronchitis
- Mucus or phlegm in the lungs or sinuses
- Regulates and strengthens the Lungs
- Stops coughing – very effective for this, due to any lung problem, including colds and flu, allergies, or asthma
- Wheezing

Lung 7 is a major point that treats coughing, wheezing, and bronchitis with cough. Acupuncture and acupressure can speed up the recovery from colds and flu by stimulating the immune system, and resolving mucus production. It is common to stop coughing within minutes of getting acupuncture on Lung 7. For colds and flu, treat Large Intestine 4 and 11, Stomach 36 and 40. I would recommend treatment at least every two hours. Acupressure is effective on this point.

## Lung 9

At the thumb side of the wrist crease, in the depression on the lateral side of the radial artery.

## Functions and Common Usage

This point strengthens the lungs and resolves mucus in the lungs. It regulates lung function to treat cough, asthma, wheezing, and difficult breathing.

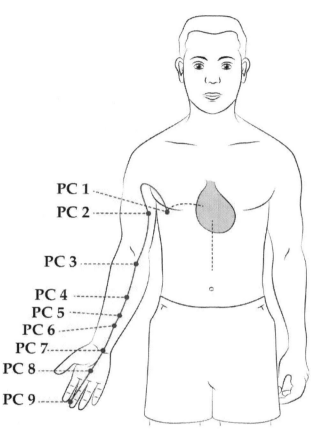

PC 1
PC 2
PC 3
PC 4
PC 5
PC 6
PC 7
PC 8
PC 9

**Pericardium Meridian**

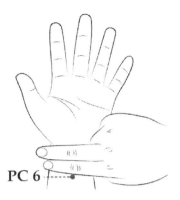

PC 6

## Pericardium 6

Located 2 cun above the wrist crease, between the tendons in the middle of the forearm.

## Functions and Common Usage

- Anxiety, calms the mind
- Calms the stomach
- Expedites and regulates lactation, per one source
- Heart Fire, which causes emotional disturbances
- Heart pounding, when you feel your heart beating
- Heart rhythm disorders (consider Heart 5 also)
- Hiccups, it relaxes the diaphragm
- Improves chest circulation to treat difficult breathing
- Inability to speak or loss of memory after a stroke
- Insomnia
- Nausea during pregnancy, including morning sickness
- Palpitations (when you feel your heart beating)
- Regulates the Heart
- Regulates the stomach to treat nausea and vomiting

- Relieves heart pain, angina
- Restores healthy circulation in the chest
- Strengthens the Heart
- Very calming emotionally, often combined with Heart 7 to treat anxiety

This point regulates the stomach, as well as the heart, and the entire chest. It is used to treat anxiety, insomnia, emotional disorders, chest pain, palpitations, and chest fullness.

## Clinical Notes

This point is one of the most important points on the body. Acupressure is very effective on this point, there are wrist bands for pregnant women to use for morning sickness that apply gentle pressure to this point all day to relieve nausea. I would recommend alternating wrists for this. The points will not be as responsive if they are continually stimulated. You can put the wrist band on one arm for the day or as needed, then switch to the other arm the next day. Acupuncture is very effective to treat the causes of morning sickness.

## Insomnia Point

Acupressure done with a magnetic pellet is very effective to treat insomnia. Just place the magnetic pellet on the point an hour or so before bed, and take it off in the morning. It will help you get to sleep, and stay asleep all night.

Pericardium 6 is famous for treating nausea due to any cause, it regulates the Stomach. It opens the chest to relieve chest pain. Be sure to seek qualified care for any chest pain.

Chest pain can be caused by many things, including heart attacks, hiatal hernia, acid reflux, and other digestive issues.

It is sometimes difficult to diagnose the cause of chest pain, because it has so many possible causes. This point relieves chest pain, because it regulates the entire chest. Knowing the cause is not always necessary with acupressure. You can just use the points and allow your body to regulate itself.

If you are taking a boat trip, you can put a magnetic pellet on Pericardium 6 to prevent seasickness.

Please note that this point is located 2 cun above the wrist crease. This is two fingers. If you see an image of three fingers being used to measure it, the last knuckle on the three fingers should be used, not the biggest part of the fingers. There are many images online that are incorrect. It can be tricky to measure. You need to use the patient's fingers to measure. The wrist and hand have to be held at the same level, or the point will be located in a different place.

The easiest way to locate Pericardium 6 is to just use two fingers at the largest knuckles. If you bend your hand back at the wrist, the point location will be slightly off. If you measure the point correctly, mark the spot with a pen, then tilt your hand back, you will see it is in a different location.

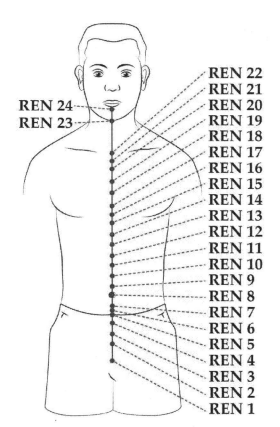

**Ren Meridian - Conception Vessel**

The Ren meridian is also called the Conception Vessel. The abbreviation for Conception Vessel is CV, so you will see this meridian under both those names.

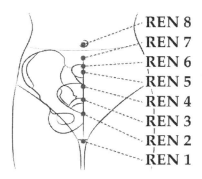

## Ren 6

Located 1.5 cun below the navel, on the midline.

### Functions and Common Usage

- Kidney stones
- Rectal prolapse
- Regulates the Ren meridian
- Regulates urination
- Restores collapsed Yin or Yang
- Strengthens the kidneys
- Tonifies Qi and Yang to treat fatigue
- Uterine prolapse

Ren 6 is a major point. It is used to improve energy levels, as well as treat prolapse of the uterus, rectum, and vagina. A prolapse is when the organ slips down from its normal position. In Chinese medicine theory, organ prolapse is caused by weak energy levels that cause your body to not be able to hold organs in their proper locations. Chinese herbs are often used for this also. There are herbal formulas that not only strongly boost energy, but that lift the energy to treat prolapsed organs. Chinese tonic herbs are very effective to restore energy levels.

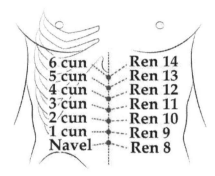

**Ren 12**
Located 4 cun above the navel, on the midline.

**Functions and Common Usage**
- Abdominal pain
- Acid reflux
- Burning pain in the throat and esophagus from acid reflux
- Clears Stomach Fire and heat, which is an inflammation of the stomach
- Descends Stomach Qi

- Gastritis
- Hiccups
- Regulates digestion
- Strengthens the Spleen and Stomach to improve digestion
- Treats stagnant digestion
- Ulcers
- Undigested food in the stool
- Vomiting

Ren 12 is a major point to regulate digestion. The stomach is supposed to digest food and send it to the small intestine. If it gets stuck in the stomach and it cannot be digested, it can cause acid reflux, hiatal hernia, and vomiting. Stomach Fire symptoms are similar to gastritis. The stomach feels like it is on fire. Ren 12 clears that type of inflammation.

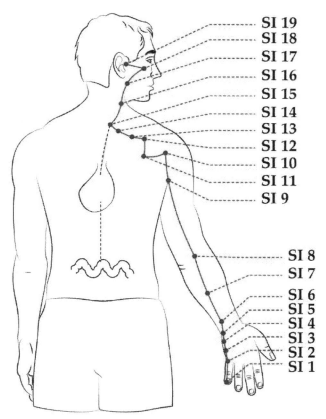

SI 19
SI 18
SI 17
SI 16
SI 15
SI 14
SI 13
SI 12
SI 10
SI 11
SI 9

SI 8
SI 7
SI 6
SI 5
SI 4
SI 3
SI 2
SI 1

**Small Intestine Meridian**

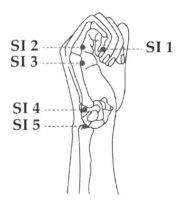

## Small Intestine 3

At the fifth metacarpophalangeal joint (knuckle), locate with the hand in a loose fist.

## Functions and Common Usage

- Calms the mind
- Conjunctivitis
- Deafness
- Elbow pain
- Epilepsy
- Eye disorders such as pain, redness, and swelling
- Finger pain
- Hand pain
- Headache on the occiput, or the base of the skull
- Lower back and sacrum pain
- Manic depression, calms the mind
- Neck pain or stiffness
- Regulates the spine
- Relaxes the muscles
- Shoulder pain
- Stiff neck

- Tinnitus
- Upper back pain or stiffness
- Whiplash

Small Intestine 3 is called the "Stiff Neck Point" by many acupuncturists. The indication of manic depression is from the diagnosis of "phlegm heat." This is how Chinese medicine treats emotional disorders. Each emotional imbalance has a root cause, which has a specific diagnosis in Chinese medicine terms. Acupuncture and herbs can be used to treat the underlying imbalance, which can help treat emotional issues that are caused by that imbalance. The diagnosis is made using Chinese medicine diagnosis, not the Western diagnosis.

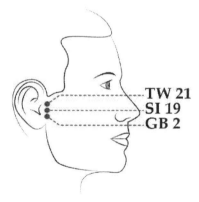

**Small Intestine 19**
Located in front of the ear tragus, and behind the condyloid process of the jawbone. The depression is more obvious when the mouth is open.

**Functions and Common Usage**

- Deafness
- Ear discharge
- Ear inflammation
- Headache due to ear issues
- Tinnitus
- Treats the ears
- Vertigo due to ear problems

As you can see in the image, Small Intestine 19 is located in front of the ear, it strongly promotes improved circulation in the ear, so ear disorders can be resolved. Any disorder caused by ear blockage will benefit from improving circulation in the ear.

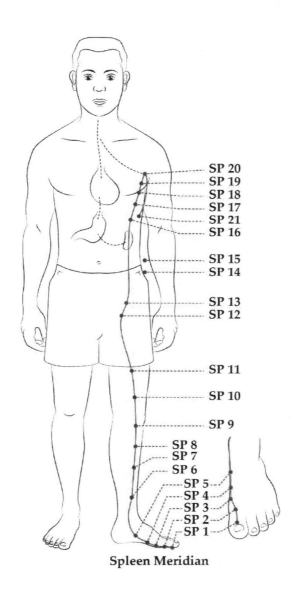

**Spleen Meridian**

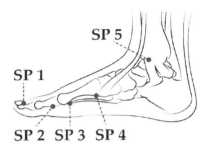

## Spleen 3
Located below the head of the first foot bone, by the big toe.

### Functions and Common Usage
- Abdominal distension
- Edema
- Fatigue
- Improves digestion
- Nausea
- Strengthens and regulates the Spleen and Stomach
- Toe pain
- Vomiting

Spleen 3 improves digestion and treats edema, which is the retention of excess fluid. It improves energy levels by improving digestion, and the ability to remove excess fluid in the body, which can cause fatigue.

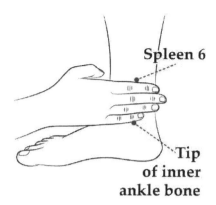

**Spleen 6**
**of inner**
**ankle bone**

**Spleen 6**
Located on the inside of the leg, 3 cun above the tip of the medial malleolus, behind the tibia bone. Locate with your whole hand on the tip of the ankle bone. You can easily locate the point by pressing on the area to find the back of the bone.

**Functions and Common Usage**
- Abdominal distention, bloating in the abdomen
- Amenorrhea – lack of menstruation
- Anemia, blood deficiency in Chinese medicine
- Anxiety
- Balances hormones
- Blurred vision from a Blood deficiency
- Calms the mind
- Dizziness from a Blood deficiency
- Edema, or retention of excess fluid
- Foot paralysis
- Genital pain
- Headache
- Hernia

- High blood pressure that is caused by Kidney deficiency
- Impotence
- Incontinence (combine with Kidney 3, 6, 7)
- Infertility
- Insomnia
- Labor induction, this point should not be used during pregnancy due to its possible effect on inducing labor
- Nourishes the Blood and Yin
- Painful urination
- Promotes urination, causes the body to excrete excess fluid
- Regulates menstruation
- Regulates the blood when it is stagnant, or blood circulation is impaired
- Regulates the Liver
- Relieves pain on the Spleen meridian
- Skin diseases, cools the Blood to treat skin problems like eczema and hives
- Strengthens the Kidneys
- Strengthens the Spleen and Stomach
- Stress
- Urine retention, the inability to urinate
- Uterine prolapse

As you can see from this list of functions and indications, you could almost say that when in doubt, Spleen 6 should be treated. The key things to consider are that it regulates and strengthens the Spleen, Stomach, Kidneys, and the Liver. It treats ailments that have their root in an imbalance in those organs. I would say that it is a rare patient who would not benefit from having this point treated. It is very calming and it treats the underlying cause of insomnia.

Spleen 6 strengthens the Spleen to encourage the body to get rid of excess fluid. This excess fluid tends to accumulate around the ankles, and on the feet. To test for the presence of edema, press firmly on an area for about a minute. If there is an indentation left behind when you stop pressing that is a sign you are retaining fluid. People often do not notice they have this problem. Acupuncture is very effective to resolve excess fluid. If your finger leaves an indentation, it is called "pitting edema." There is a "pit" where your finger pressed.

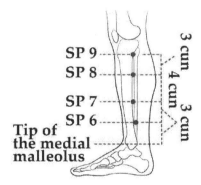

**Spleen 8**
Located 3 cun below Spleen 9, behind the crest of the tibia bone.

**Functions and Common Usage**
- Regulates the menstrual cycle
- Strengthens the Spleen

- Regulates the uterus
- Regulates Blood
- Menstrual cramps

This point can be used to treat abnormal uterine bleeding. It is also used to treat painful or irregular menstrual cycles. Menstrual problems can be caused by "stagnant blood" in the uterus. That means that the blood is not flowing properly. This point regulates the blood in the uterus to help resolve menstrual issues.

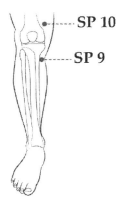

SP 10

SP 9

**Spleen 9**
Located in the depression by the knee that is at the end of the tibia bone.

**Functions and Common Usage**
- Abdominal pain
- Edema
- Genital pain
- Knee pain
- Regulates the Stomach
- Strengthens the Spleen

This point is the number one point used to treat edema, or excess fluid anywhere in the body. It encourages the body to expel excess fluid.

**SP 10**

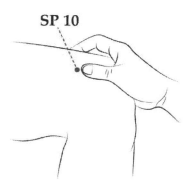

**Spleen 10**
Located 2 cun from the upper border of the kneecap. You can locate this point by cupping your hand over the kneecap. The point is located at the tip of your thumb, on the inside of the leg.

**Functions and Common Usage**
- Blood disorders
- Cools Heat in the Blood
- Eczema
- Genital itching or pain
- Hives
- Irregular menses
- Itching anywhere on the body
- Knee pain
- Painful menstruation
- Regulates Blood circulation
- Regulates Spleen Qi
- Skin disorders involving heat or inflammation

This point is called the "Sea of Blood." It regulates blood circulation. It is also a cooling point, meaning that it clears disorders that involve inflammation, especially in the skin. It is also used to treat knee pain. It restores healthy blood flow through the knee. The Stomach and Spleen meridians are often used to treat knee pain, because the Spleen meridian is located on the inside of the leg, and the Stomach meridian is on the outside of the leg. Using both of these meridians will encourage healthy blood circulation through the knee.

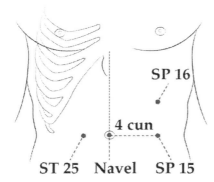

### Spleen 15
Located at the level of the navel, 4 cun lateral to the midline.

### Functions and Common Usage
- Abdominal pain
- Constipation
- Fecal incontinence
- Regulates the intestines
- Moistens the intestines

This point is used to regulate the intestines. It treats constipation, and it can be combined with other points for constipation such as Large Intestine 11. It restores the normal function of the intestines.

The expression "moistens the intestines" means that it can also treat stubborn constipation, when the stools have dried out. The longer you go without a bowel movement, the drier the stools become. Spleen 15 and Large Intestine 11 are effective to stimulate the Large Intestine, or the colon to empty. Acupressure is effective on both of these points.

Fecal incontinence is when you cannot control your bowels. There are two types of incontinence, urinary and fecal, or stool. Treating your kidneys via Kidney 3, 6, and 7 will treat urinary incontinence. Stomach 36, and Spleen 15 will treat fecal incontinence. These disorders are more common in older age, because the energy of your body naturally declines.

You can avoid incontinence by getting acupuncture to keep everything working properly. I would also suggest Chinese Kidney tonics like Cordyceps. Your acupuncturist will have much stronger Kidney tonic herbs, but Cordyceps can be purchased over the counter to strengthen the kidneys. This will also relieve fatigue.

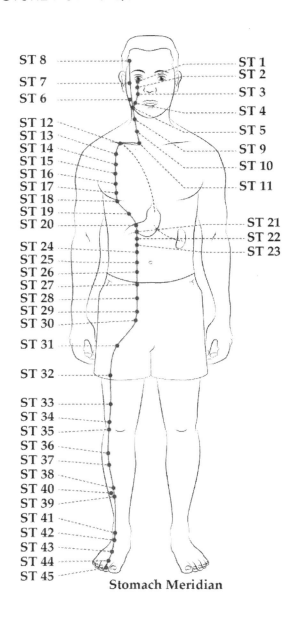

ST 8
ST 7
ST 6
ST 12
ST 13
ST 14
ST 15
ST 16
ST 17
ST 18
ST 19
ST 20
ST 24
ST 25
ST 26
ST 27
ST 28
ST 29
ST 30
ST 31
ST 32
ST 33
ST 34
ST 35
ST 36
ST 37
ST 38
ST 40
ST 39
ST 41
ST 42
ST 43
ST 44
ST 45

ST 1
ST 2
ST 3
ST 4
ST 5
ST 9
ST 10
ST 11
ST 21
ST 22
ST 23

**Stomach Meridian**

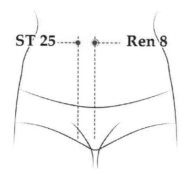

## Stomach 25
Located 2 cun lateral to the navel.

## Functions and Common Usage
- Abdominal pain
- Appendicitis
- Colitis
- Constipation
- Diarrhea
- Edema
- Intestinal abscess
- Intestinal obstruction
- Moistens and regulates the intestines to treat constipation
- Navel pain
- Pancreatitis
- Regulates digestion
- Regulates menstruation
- Regulates the intestines
- Vomiting

This point should not be used during pregnancy.

This is a major point to treat digestive disorders. It is combined with other points to regulate the intestines, and to treat both constipation and diarrhea. It improves circulation in the intestines, which regulates intestinal function. It can be used after abdominal surgery to restore normal function.

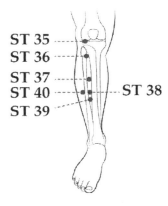

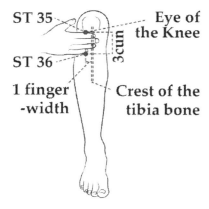

## Stomach 36
Located 3 cun below Stomach 35, and one finger width from the anterior crest of the tibia bone.

Stomach 36 can be located several ways. You can place your hand over your knee to measure the point. The index finger is placed at the level of the eyes of the knee, which are the small depressions on both sides of your kneecap. The point is just below your little finger. You can also cross reference the location by using the tibia, or calf bone.

### Functions and Common Usage
Stomach 36 is perhaps the most commonly used point in acupuncture. It has so many functions that I will separate the functions from the indications to make it easier to understand. Acupressure is effective on this point.

### Regulates and strengthens the Spleen and Stomach
- Abdominal fullness
- Abdominal pain
- Belching
- Constipation
- Diaphragm spasms
- Diarrhea
- Difficulty swallowing
- Edema, fluid retention
- Fatigue
- Gastritis
- Hiccup
- Indigestion
- Mastitis

- Nausea
- Pancreatitis
- Poor appetite
- Prolapse of organs
- Stomach pain
- Vomiting

## Regulates and strengthens the Lungs
- Asthma
- Breathing difficulty
- Cough
- Fatigue
- Immune system tonic, can be used for allergies, cold and flu, and general immune system weakness
- Shortness of breath

## Regulates and moistens the intestines
- Abdominal pain
- Appendicitis
- Constipation
- Diarrhea
- Enteritis, inflammation of the intestines
- Intestinal abscess

## Regulates and strengthens the immune system
- Allergies
- Colds and flu
- Hives

## Miscellaneous
- Anemia, helps to build blood
- Benefits lactation

- Blurred vision
- Breast abscess
- Difficulty swallowing
- Dizziness
- Hemiplegia
- High blood pressure, combine with other points to treat the underlying cause
- Knee pain, combined with other points
- Knee weakness
- Leg pain
- Leg paralysis
- Leg weakness
- Leukorrhea
- Mastitis

This point is one of the best points on the body to improve energy levels. It improves digestion, and relieves fatigue. It is called "Leg Three Miles," because the saying goes that even when you are at the point of exhaustion, you can treat this point and walk three more miles.

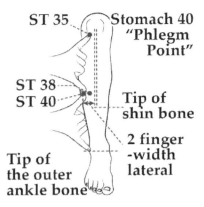

## Stomach 40

Located halfway between the eye of the knee and the lateral malleolus, or outer ankle bone. To locate place your little finger over the tip of the outer ankle bone, and the other little finger in the eye of the knee, which is the small indentation by your kneecap. The halfway point is located where your thumbs meet in the middle. The point is located at this level, 2 finger widths from your tibia or shin bone.

## Functions and Common Usage

- Asthma
- Bronchitis
- Calms the mind
- Chest or lung problems
- Chest pain from lung issues
- Cold and flu symptoms with excess mucus production
- Cough caused by excess mucus
- Constipation
- Coughing
- Dizziness

- Lower leg pain or paralysis
- Pneumonia
- Regulates the intestines
- Regulates the stomach
- Shortness of breath from mucus in the lungs
- Stomach Fire – gastritis
- Throat pain, obstruction, and swelling
- Transforms phlegm
- Wheezing
- Whooping cough

Stomach 40 is called the *Phlegm Point*. It helps to resolve phlegm, or mucus, anywhere in the body. It is helpful for colds and flu, as it resolves mucus. This point can be combined with Stomach 36, Large Intestine 4 and 11, and Lung 7. This boosts the immune system and resolves phlegm.

People often cancel their acupuncture appointments when they get a cold or flu. Getting acupuncture can help you resolve your cold or flu much faster. I once treated my dad every 2 hours and the next day he was almost symptom free. He had a horrible cough from a cold, and he needed to get well quickly, so I gave him frequent treatments. The next day he rarely coughed and was almost completely well.

When a treatment for excess mucus is given, using Stomach 40, patients often start coughing after the needles are removed. That shows that the mucus in the lungs is being resolved. Your body starts to resolve the mucus by coughing, which is how it expels it. This point can also be used to treat asthma, which is described as the retention of mucus in the lungs, obstructing normal Lung function. It should be combined with other points, and Chinese herbal medicine to treat asthma.

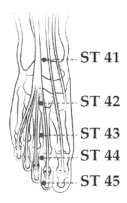

## Stomach 41
Located at the ankle, at the level of the lateral malleolus, or outside ankle bone, in the depression between the tendons.

### Functions and Common Usage
- Ankle pain
- Foot drop
- Foot pain
- Headache on the forehead, caused by Stomach issues
- Lower leg pain, atrophy, or stiffness
- Stomach Fire or gastritis

This point is commonly used to restore normal function to the foot, to treat foot pain, or toe pain.

- Clears heat in the Stomach meridian
- Foot pain or weakness
- Facial paralysis or swelling

- Foot atrophy

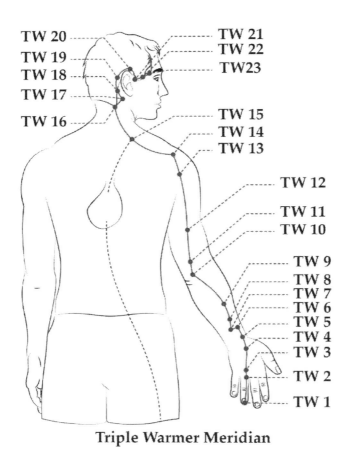

TW 20
TW 19
TW 18
TW 17
TW 16

TW 21
TW 22
TW23

TW 15
TW 14
TW 13

TW 12

TW 11
TW 10

TW 9
TW 8
TW 7
TW 6
TW 5
TW 4
TW 3

TW 2

TW 1

**Triple Warmer Meridian**

The Triple Warmer meridian is also called the San Jiao meridian. The concept of a Triple Warmer is the ancient way of looking at energy production in the body. There are three warmers, the upper, middle, and lower burners.

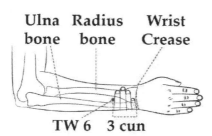

**Triple Warmer 6**
Located 3 cun from the wrist crease, in the depression between the radius and ulna bone.

**Functions and Common Usage**
- Benefits the voice
- Constipation
- Opens the intestines
- Sudden loss of voice
- Throat pain
- Tinnitus

Triple Warmer 6 resolves stagnation and opens the intestines. Triple Warmer 6 is used for severe constipation, in combination with other points like Large Intestine 11, and Stomach 36. The points chosen depend on the underlying cause of the problem.

# Extra Points

These points are listed in Chinese first, because they do not have numbers that are commonly used. In most cases the English translation is placed first on the image, but most acupuncturists refer to the points by the Chinese name. These points are called "extra points" because they are in most cases not located on a meridian.

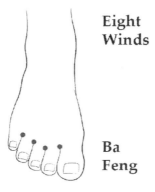

Eight
Winds

Ba
Feng

**Ba Feng – Eight Winds**
On the top of the foot, between the toes, on the web margins. There are eight points in total.

**Functions and Common Usage**
Treat foot pain, and headaches. The Ba Feng points are excellent to treat diabetic neuropathy. They work by restoring normal circulation in the feet.

**Clinical Notes**
Ba Feng are effective to restore healthy circulation in the feet. I use them for diabetic neuropathy or any type of nerve

problem in the feet. They are very effective for foot numbness. Patients do not mind them at first, until the nerves wake up and start working again, then they can be sensitive and painful. Once they start to hurt, you know the nerves are working better and you don't need the points as much.

I would also consider using Ba Feng to treat leg problems after a stroke. Treating the ends of the feet is very effective to restore normal nerve function. Acupuncture is preferred, but any type of acupressure will help. Using a massager in this area, or just massaging the points with your fingers helps.

**Eight Pathogens**

**Ba Xie**

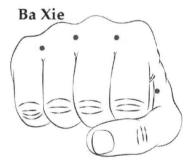

### Ba Xie – Eight Pathogens
On the top of the hand, at the junction of the white and red skin of the hand webs. Eight points in all.

### Functions and Common Usage
These points treat numbness, stiffness, and pain in the fingers and hand.

## Clinical Notes

They are very effective to improve blood flow to the hand and treat and type of hand problem. They also can be used to treat nerve problems. By stimulating the nerves, they regulate nerve function. (When nerves are damaged they tend to misfire. Shooting pains and the loss of control of the hands can be caused by damaged nerves. When the hands are numb, there is a lack of circulation. Stimulating these points encourages restored function). These points correspond to Ba Feng, located between the toes. They both are helpful for nerve diseases.

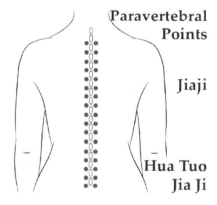

## Hua Tuo Jia Ji – Paravertebral Points

A group of 34 points on both sides of the spine, located .5 cun lateral to the lower border of each spinous process. The points run from the first thoracic vertebrae, to the fifth lumbar vertebrae. These points are commonly called the Jiaji points.

**Functions and Common Usage**
These points can be used to regulate the spinal nerves. They are most commonly used to treat back pain. They strongly stimulate nerve function in the spine to relieve pain, and restore healthy function.

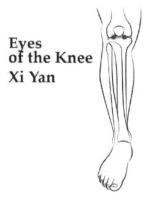

Eyes
of the Knee
Xi Yan

**Xi Yan – Eyes of the Knee**
Two points on either side of the patellar ligament. Located in the eyes of the knee, which are located by the kneecap.

**Functions and Common Usage**
Treats pain in the knee joint, difficulty moving the knee, and weak knees. This point is commonly combined with other points around the knee joint like He Ding, ST 34, ST 36, SP 9, and SP 10.

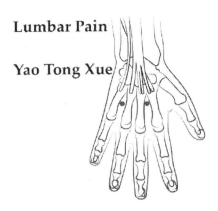

## Yao Tong Xue – Lumbar Pain Points

On the top of the hand, between the second and third hand bones, and between the fourth and fifth hand bones. There are two points on each hand.

## Functions and Common Usage

Used for lower back pain.

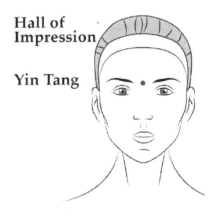

## Yin Tang – Hall of Impression, or Spirit Gate
Midway between the medial ends of the two eyebrows.

## Functions and Common Usage
Calms the mind, benefits the nose, treats insomnia, and nasal congestion.  This point is very effective to treat insomnia, and it is very calming.

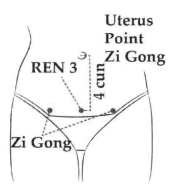

## Zi Gong – Uterus Point, or Palace of the Child
Three cun lateral to Ren 3.  Located 4 cun below the navel and 1 cun above the pubic bone.

## Functions and Common Usage
Zi Gong regulates menstruation.  It treats prolapse of the uterus, infertility, and abnormal uterine bleeding.  This point is used a lot to treat infertility.  It improves blood flow in the pelvis, and it has been shown to even unblock fallopian tubes in some cases.

## How Acupuncture Improves Fertility

- Restores healthy blood flow in the pelvis
- Improve the Kidneys, which is how Chinese medicine treats hormonal imbalances
- Regulates the Liver, which regulates the hormones
- Restores complete health, which is necessary for healthy fertility

Acupuncture and Chinese herbal medicine should be given to both the male and female. Acupuncture restores health, it does not treat infertility as a separate entity. It restores health, so your body can function normally. Common patterns that are seen in infertility patients are:

- Liver Qi stagnation
- Kidney deficiency
- Blood stagnation

In addition to helping improve the odds of conception, acupuncture can also be used to improve the mother's health during pregnancy. If the mother gets acupuncture during her pregnancy, her baby is often very calm. The acupuncture treats and calms the baby, as it treats the mother. These babies are called *Acupuncture Babies*. It is a well-known phenomenon that *Acupuncture Babies* are very calm and cry less than other babies.

# Resources

I used multiple sources for the images in this book. I cross-referenced several books and chose the most commonly used locations and functions of each point.

*A Manual of Acupuncture* by Peter Deadman, Mazin Al-Khafaji and Kevin Baker. This is the book acupuncture students use to learn point locations in school.

*Acupuncture Points Images and Functions*, by Arnie Lade. This book does not have all the points, and it does not have point images. It is an extremely good reference for a broad range of point functions.

*Acupuncture A Comprehensive Text*, Shanghai College of Traditional Medicine, by John O'Connor and Dan Bensky. This is called simply the "Shanghai Book" by most acupuncturists. It is a reference book for many acupuncture students.

*The Foundations of Chinese Medicine* by Giovanni Maciocia. This is the first year text for acupuncture students. It explains Chinese medicine diagnosis and Chinese medicine theory.

*The Practice of Chinese Medicine* by Giovanni Maciocia. This is the second year book for acupuncture students. Dozens of diseases are explained in Chinese medicine terms. It explains how to diagnose and treat diseases, which acupuncture points to use, and which herbal formulas to use.

# Index

## About the Author

Deborah Bleecker is a Licensed Acupuncturist, and has a Master of Science degree in Oriental Medicine. A degree in Oriental Medicine is a combination of acupuncture, and Chinese herbal medicine. This is a complete system of medicine that has been used for thousands of years.

She was injured on the job in 1994 and lived with chronic pain until she decided she would have to find her own answers to her health problems. Medical doctors told her that her pain was incurable, but she was able to recover with the help of acupuncture and Chinese herbs.

She can be reached at deborahbleecker@gmail.com, and her website is www.acupunctureexplained..com.

# Reviews

If you like this book, please consider leaving a review online. Most readers do not even consider buying a book unless it has at least 100 reviews. The length of the review does not matter, anything you can do is greatly appreciated.

Thank you.

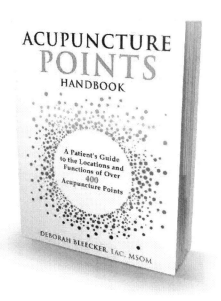

*Acupuncture Points Handbook* includes information on the locations and functions of over 400 acupuncture points.

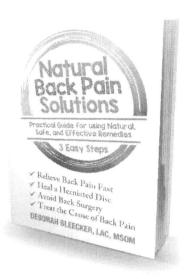

*Natural Back Pain Solutions* includes dozens of natural remedies for back pain. After 20 years of treating back pain as an acupuncturist, I have compiled the best back pain remedies you can buy. You can effectively treat your own back pain with the remedies in this book.

Supplement recommendations, as well as information on the best acupressure points for back pain are included. There are many natural options for pain relief. These remedies are safe, and very effective.

Printed in Poland
by Amazon Fulfillment
Poland Sp. z o.o., Wrocław

50611195R00078